NATHALIE WOODS

Nature's Secret

TO BEAUTIFUL SKIN

**35 DIY Organic Skincare Recipes
for a Natural and Radiant Glow**

CONTENTS

CONTENTS

INTRODUCTION

DIY natural skincare is a great way to take care of your skin using only natural, safe and effective ingredients.

These recipes are made with simple, easy-to-find ingredients that you can use to create your own skincare products at home.

These recipes are designed to be gentle and nourishing for all skin types, and will help you achieve a healthy, radiant complexion.

Whether you're looking for a new face mask, exfoliating scrub, or moisturizer, these recipes will provide you with a variety of options to suit your individual skincare needs.

These recipes are also a great way to save money and reduce your environmental impact by avoiding commercially-produced skincare products that are often filled with synthetic ingredients and packaging.

By using natural skincare products, you are not only taking care of your skin, but you are also supporting the environment.

With these 35 recipes, you'll have all the tools you need to create a complete natural skincare routine, tailored to your individual needs.

Keep in mind that these are just suggestions and you can always play around with the quantity of the ingredients according to your preference and skin type.

It's always recommended to do a patch test before using any new ingredients on your skin, some people may have allergies or sensitivity to certain ingredients.

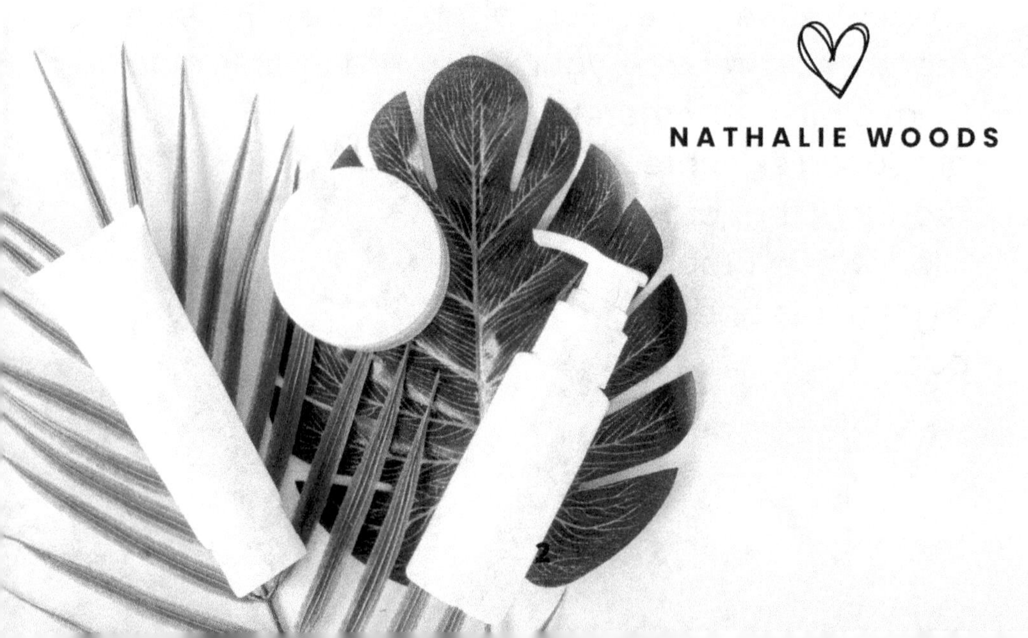

NATHALIE WOODS

Honey & Turmeric Face Mask

- Mix 2 tablespoons of honey with 1 teaspoon of turmeric powder.

- Apply the mixture to your face and leave on for 15-20 minutes before rinsing off.

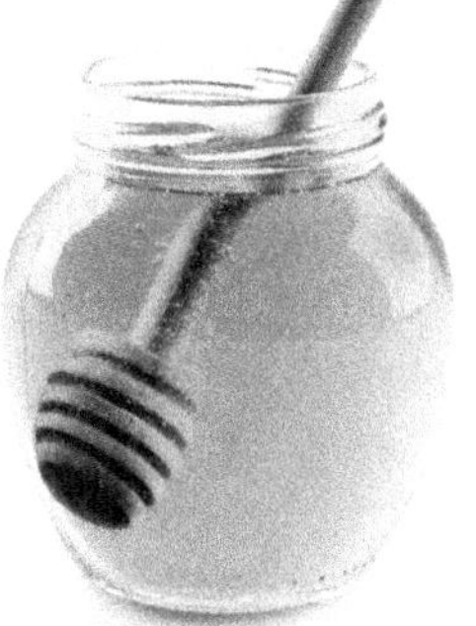

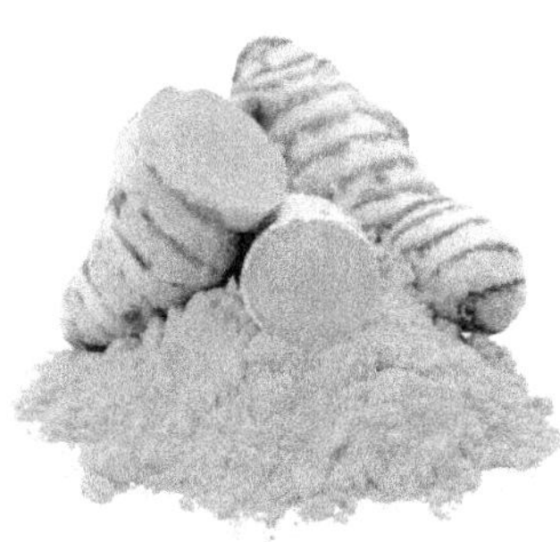

HONEY:

- Deeply Moisturizes and Hydrates the Skin.
- Diminishes the Signs of Premature Aging.
- An Effective Pore Cleanser and Gentle Exfoliator.
- Lightens Scars and Hyperpigmentation.
- Fights Acne and Breakouts.
- Relieves Sunburn.

TURMERIC:

- Could Help Heal Acne.
- Lightens Hyperpigmentation.
- Deals With Dull Skin.
- Reduces Dark Circles.
- Protects Against Environmental Damage.
- Prevents Premature Aging.
- Could Help Psoriasis and Eczema.

Oatmeal & Yogurt Exfoliating Mask

- Mix 1/2 cup of oatmeal with 1/4 cup of plain yogurt.

- Apply the mixture to your face and gently massage in circular motions for 2-3 minutes before rinsing off.

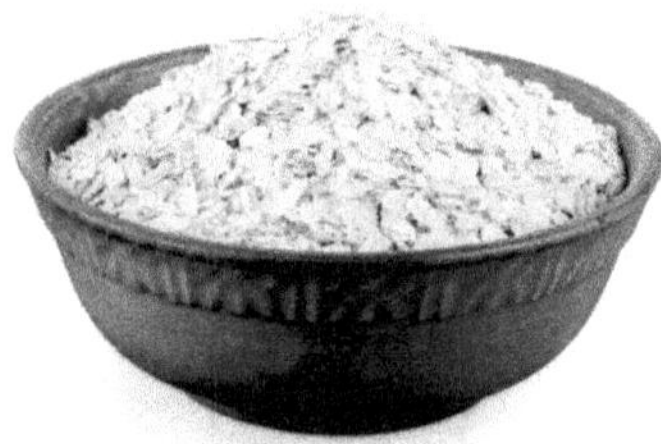 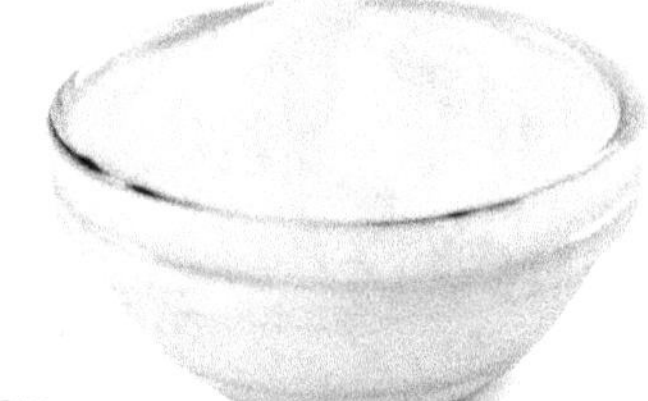

OATMEAL:

- Soothes irritated skin.
- Reduces inflammation.
- Retains moisture.
- Gentle exfoliant.
- Removes dead skin cells.
- High in antioxidants.
- Anti-inflammatory properties.
- Protects the skin from damage caused by free radicals.
- Natural cleanser.
- Removes impurities and excess oil from the skin.

YOGURT:

- Moisturizes the skin.
- Contains lactic acid, which acts as a mild exfoliant.
- Reduces the appearance of fine lines and wrinkles.
- Brightens the skin.
- Contains vitamins and minerals that are beneficial for the skin.
- Can help to reduce inflammation.
- Can help to reduce redness.

Banana & Avocado Moisturizer

- Mash 1/2 a ripe banana and 1/4 of an avocado together.

- Apply the mixture to your face and leave on for 15-20 minutes before rinsing off.

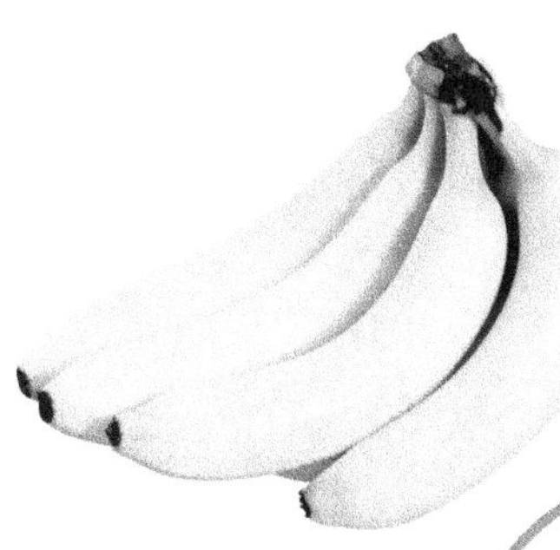

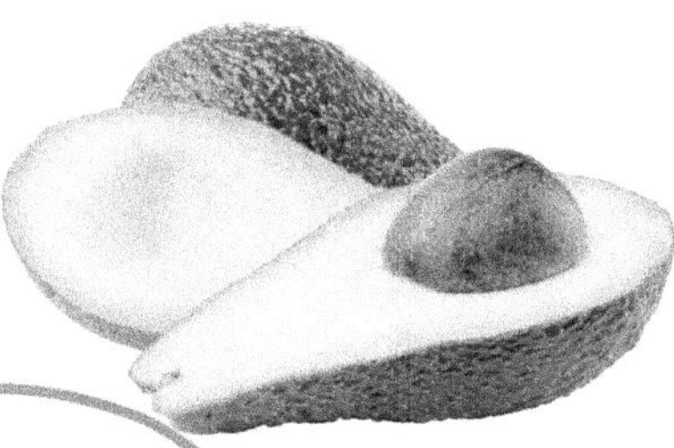

BANANA :

- Moisturizes dry skin.
- Protect the skin from damage caused by free radicals.
- Help to keep the skin firm and elastic.
- Helps to reduce the appearance of wrinkles and fine lines.
- Help to soothe sunburned skin.
- Help to reduce the appearance of acne and blemishes.

AVOCADO :

- Reduce the appearance of wrinkles and fine lines.
- Soothe sunburned skin.
- Reduce the appearance of acne and blemishes.
- Can help to lighten age spots and other forms of hyperpigmentation.
- Improve the overall texture and tone of the skin.
- Can be used as a natural exfoliant to remove dead skin cells.

Coconut Oil & Sugar Lip Scrub

- Mix 1 tablespoon of coconut oil with 1 tablespoon of sugar.

- Gently massage the mixture onto your lips in circular motions, then wipe off with a warm, damp cloth.

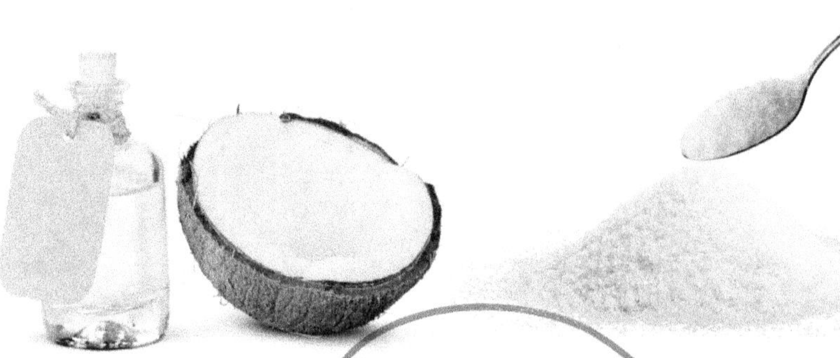

COCONUT OIL :

- Defending Skin from Damaging Microorganisms.
- Coconut Oil for Dry Skin is Highly Moisturising.
- It Can Help to Treat Acne.
- It Can Support Healing.
- It Can Help to Reduce Inflammation.
- It Contributes to a More Even Skin Tone.
- It can Help to Reduce Signs of Ageing Skin.

SUGAR :

- Good for retaining and absorbing moisture in your skin.
- Helps in making your skin smooth, soft and plumpy.
- Hydrating your skin from within by clearing the dead cells.
- Helps in removing the dead skin cells effectively.
- Clearing the skin and enhancing your complexion.

Green Tea and Lemon Toner

- Brew a cup of green tea and let it cool.

- Mix 1/4 cup of the tea with 1 tablespoon of freshly squeezed lemon juice.

- Apply the mixture to your face with a cotton ball or pad.

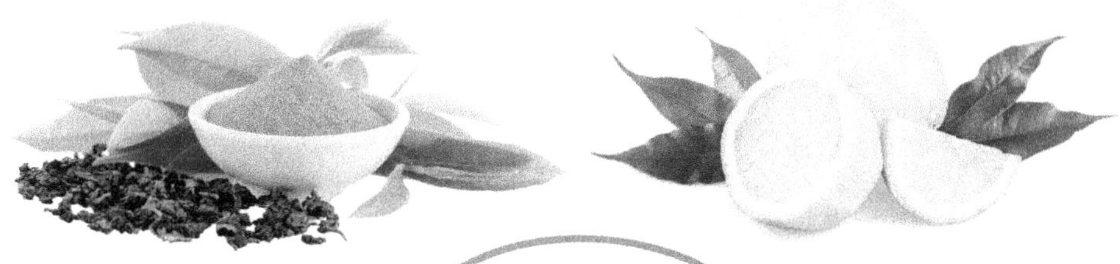

GREEN TEA :

- Fights skin cancer by promoting DNA repair.
- It has powerful anti-inflammatory properties.
- It is a powerful antibacterial agent for treating acne and unclogging pores.
- It is chock full of vitamin B2 and vitamin E, both essential for skin health.
- Help shrink blood vessels around the eyes for treating puffy eyes and dark circles.

LEMON :

- The citric acid found in lemon juice brightens your skin, making it look more youthful and radiant.
- An amazing home remedy for dark spots and acne scars.
- Lemon has antifungal and antimicrobial properties.
- Lemon juice can help prevent blemishes and blackheads.
- Lemons fight wrinkles and other signs of ageing.

Aloe Vera & Vitamin E Face Seru

- Mix 1/4 cup of aloe vera gel with 1 tablespoon of vitamin E oil.

- Apply the mixture to your face, focusing on areas of dryness or wrinkles.

ALOE VERA :

- Helps soothe sunburn.
- Helps to moisturize the skin.
- Boosts healing of wounds.
- Fights skin-ageing.
- Reduces infection and acne.
- Lightens blemishes on the face.
- Fading Dark Spots and Stretch Marks
- It may help reduce stretch marks

VITAMIN E :

- Moisturizing skin.
- Wound healing.
- Skin cancer prevention.
- Preventing or treating fine lines and wrinkles.
- Vitamin E may alleviate the dryness, itching, and flaking associated with eczema, or atopic dermatitis.
- Preventing or minimizing the appearance of scars.

Yogurt & Honey Face Cleanser

- Mix 1/4 cup of plain yogurt with 1 tablespoon of honey.

- Apply the mixture to your face and massage in circular motions for 1-2 minutes before rinsing off.

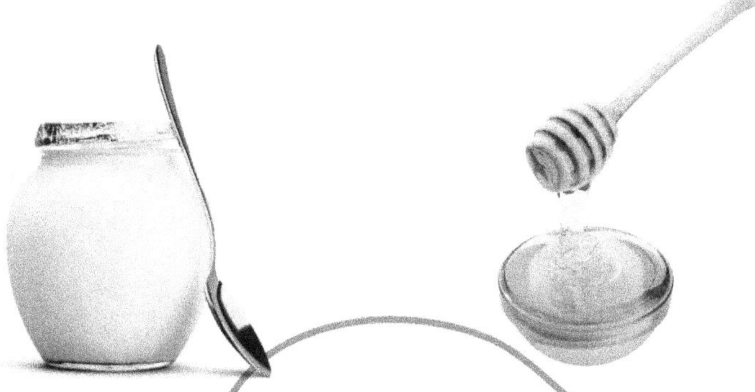

YOGURT :

- UV ray protection.
- Reduces the signs of skin aging.
- Evens skin tone.
- Fades Blemishes And Pigmentation.
- Reduces Dark Circles.
- Treats Skin Infections.
- Soothes Sunburns.

HONEY :

- Honey can help to brighten the skin, giving it a more even and radiant appearance.
- Using it to add a touch of natural glow on the face tops the chart.
- Rich in antioxidants, vitamins and minerals that can nourish the skin and boost collagen production.

Sugar & Olive Oil Body Scrub

- Mix 1/2 cup of sugar with 1/4 cup of olive oil.

- Use the mixture to gently exfoliate your skin in the shower.

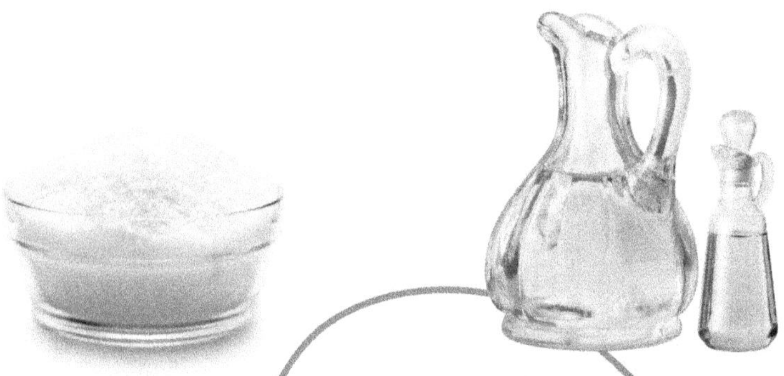

SUGAR :

- Sugar can help to stimulate blood flow, which can improve the overall health and appearance of the skin.
- Sugar contains glycolic acid, which can help to reduce the appearance of fine lines and wrinkles.
- The glycolic acid found in sugar can help to unclog pores and prevent new breakouts from forming.

OLIVE OIL :

- Olive oil is a natural emollient, which can help to keep the skin moisturized and soft.
- Olive oil can help to heal dry, cracked, or irritated skin.
- Olive oil can provide a barrier that protects the skin from environmental factors such as pollution and UV rays.

Rose Water & Glycerin Moisturizer

- Mix 1/4 cup of rose water with 1 tablespoon of glycerin.

- Apply the mixture to your face, focusing on areas of dryness.

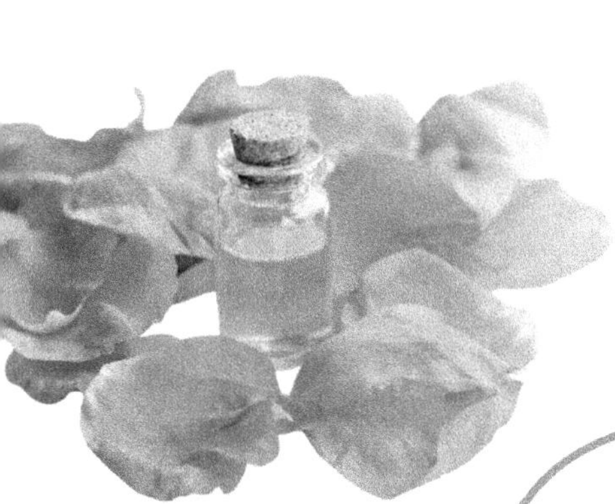

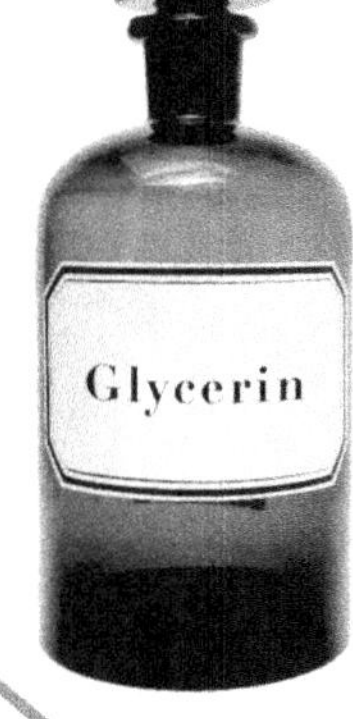

ROSE WATER :

- Rose water is a natural astringent and can help to hydrate and moisturize the skin.
- Rose water has a pleasant and refreshing scent that can leave the skin smelling nice.
- Rose water can be used as a cleanser to remove dirt, oil, and impurities from the skin.
- Rose water can help to balance the pH of the skin and tighten pores.

GLYCERIN :

- Glycerin can help to heal dry, cracked, or irritated skin.
- Glycerin is rich in antioxidants, which can help to nourish the skin and protect it from damage.
- Glycerin is a natural humectant, which means it attracts water to the skin and helps to keep it moisturized.

Lemon & Sugar Foot Scrub

- Mix 1/4 cup of sugar with 1 tablespoon of freshly squeezed lemon juice.

- Use the mixture to gently exfoliate your feet in the shower.

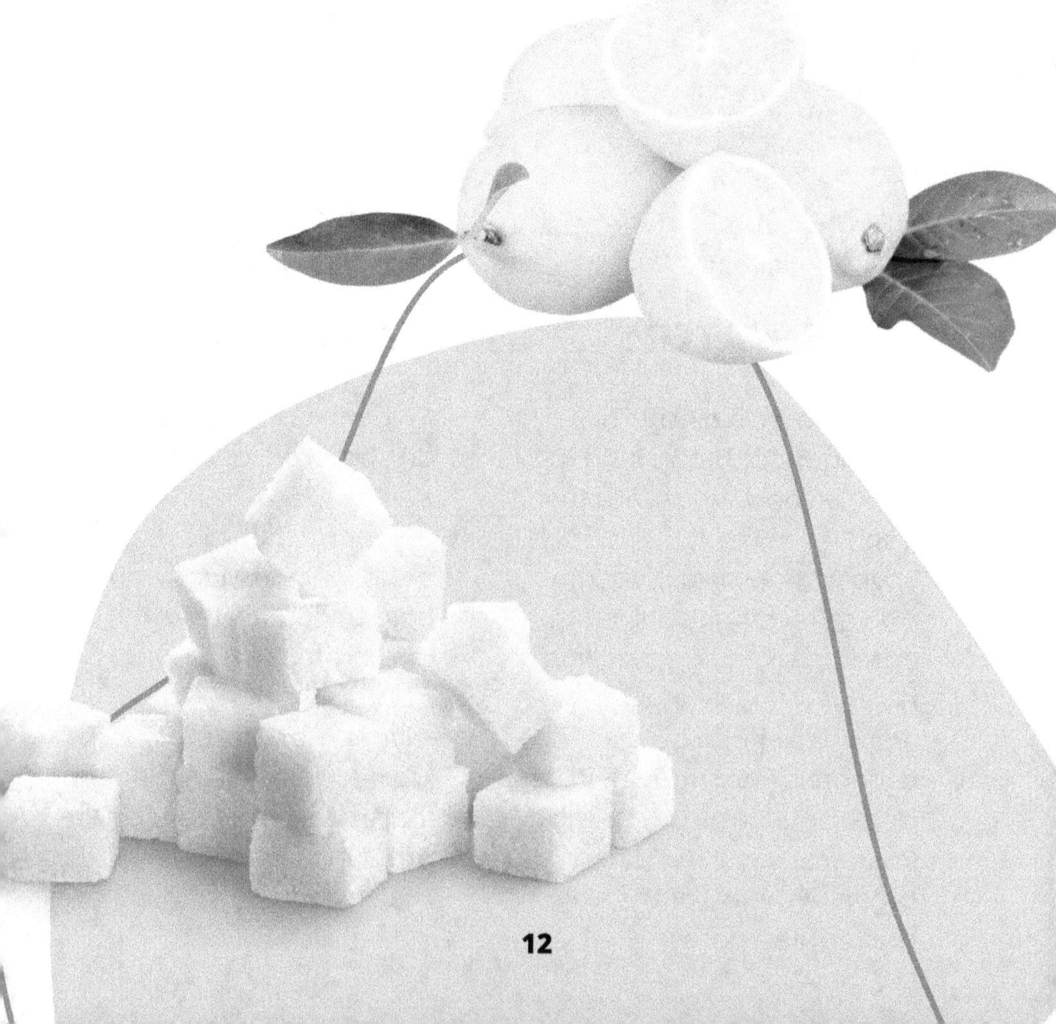

Egg White & Lemon Juice Facial Mask

- Mix 1/4 cup of sugar with 1 tablespoon of freshly squeezed lemon juice.

- Use the mixture to gently exfoliate your feet in the shower.

EGG WHITE :

- Egg whites contain proteins that can help to tighten and firm the skin.
- Egg whites can help to control excess oil production in the skin, making it less prone to acne and breakouts.
- Egg whites can help to brighten the skin, giving it a more even and radiant appearance.
- whites have anti-inflammatory properties that can help to soothe irritated or sensitive skin.

Yogurt & Oats Face Mask

- Mix 1/4 cup of plain yogurt with 1/4 cup of rolled oats.

- Apply the mixture to your face and leave on for 15-20 minutes before rinsing off.

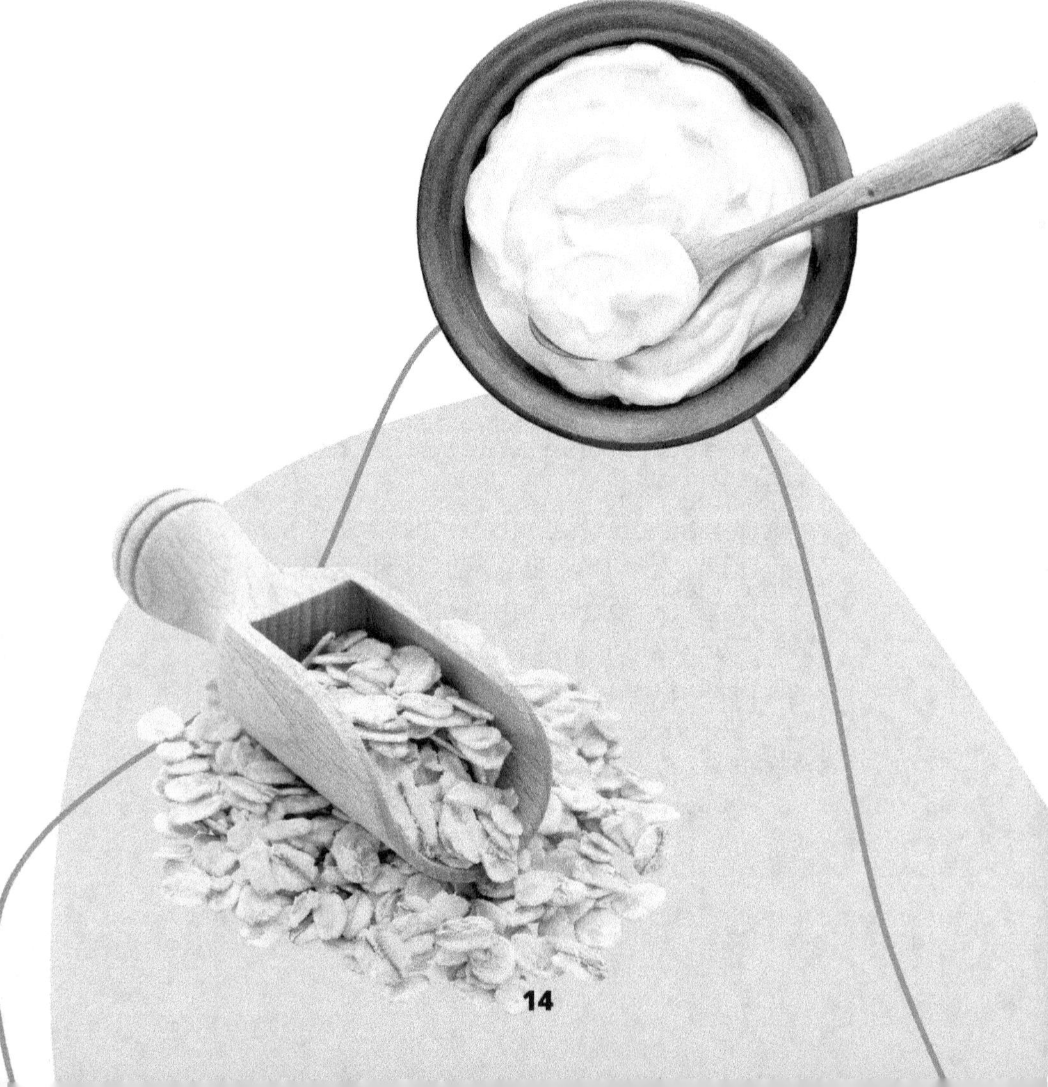

Honey & Cinnamon Acne Mask

- Mix 1 tablespoon of honey with 1 teaspoon of cinnamon powder.

- Apply the mixture to your face and leave on for 15-20 minutes before rinsing off.

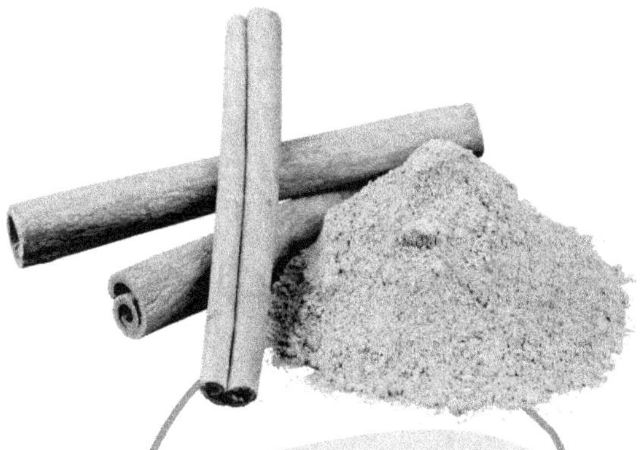

Cinnamon :

- Cinnamon contains anti-inflammatory properties which can help reduce redness and irritation.
- Cinnamon has antimicrobial properties that can help to fight acne and prevent new breakouts from forming.
- Cinnamon can help to stimulate blood flow, which can improve the overall health and appearance of the skin.
- Cinnamon can be used as a gentle exfoliant, helping to remove dead skin cells and reveal brighter, smoother skin.

Coconut Oil & Sea Salt Body Scrub

- Mix 1/4 cup of coconut oil with 1/4 cup of sea salt

- Use the mixture to gently exfoliate your skin in the shower.

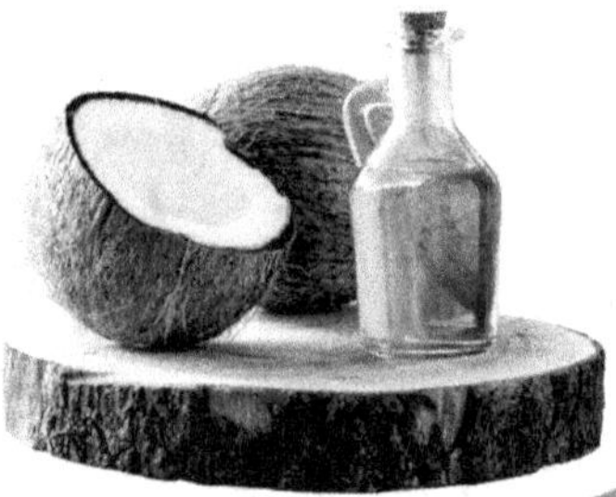

COCONUT OIL :

- Coconut oil is a natural emollient, which can help to keep the skin moisturized and soft.
- Coconut oil can help to heal dry, cracked, or irritated skin.
- Help to protect the skin from damage and reduce the appearance of fine lines and wrinkles.
- Coconut oil can help to brighten the skin, giving it a more even and radiant appearance.

SEA SALT :

- Natural exfoliant that can help to remove dead skin cells and reveal brighter, smoother skin.
- Sea salt contains minerals that can help to detoxify the skin and remove impurities.
- Sea salt can help to stimulate blood flow, which can improve the overall health and appearance of the skin.

Aloe Vera & Tea Tree Oil Spot Treatment

- Mix 1 tablespoon of aloe vera gel with 1 drop of tea tree oil.

- Apply the mixture to any blemishes on your skin.

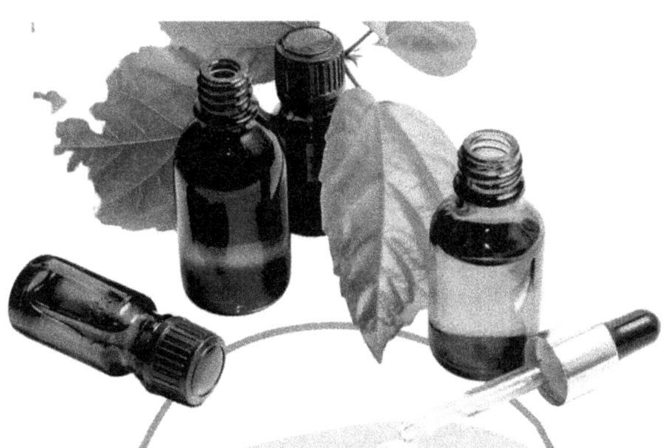

TEA TREE OIL :

- Tea tree oil may help relieve inflamed skin.
- Tea tree oil may also help reduce itchy skin.
- Tea tree oil may help speed up wound healing.
- Anti-inflammatory
- Anti-fungal
- Antiseptic

Yogurt & Blueberry Face Mask

- Mix 1/4 cup of plain yogurt with 1/4 cup of mashed blueberries.

- Apply the mixture to your face and leave on for 15-20 minutes before rinsing off.

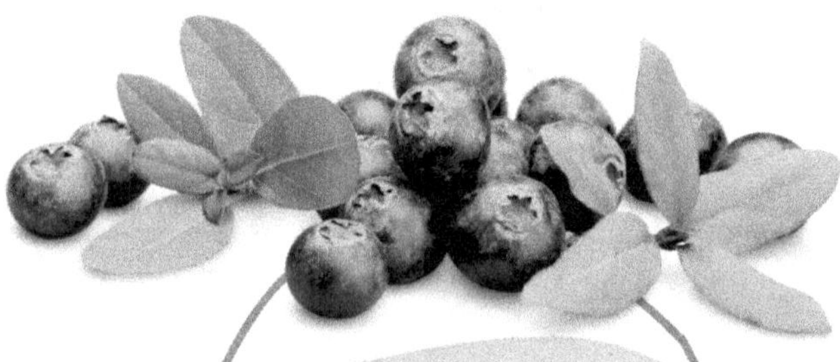

BLUEBERRY :

- Rich in antioxidants, which can protect the skin from damage caused by free radicals.
- May improve skin elasticity.
- May reduce inflammation.
- Blueberries contain a compound called "delphinidin" which can help lighten under eye dark circles.
- May help to reduce the appearance of fine lines and wrinkles.
- Blueberries are rich in Vitamin C, which can help to hydrate the skin and improve its overall appearance.

Avocado & Honey Hair Mask

- Mix 1/2 a ripe avocado with 2 tablespoons of honey.

- Apply the mixture to your hair and leave on for 30 minutes before rinsing off.

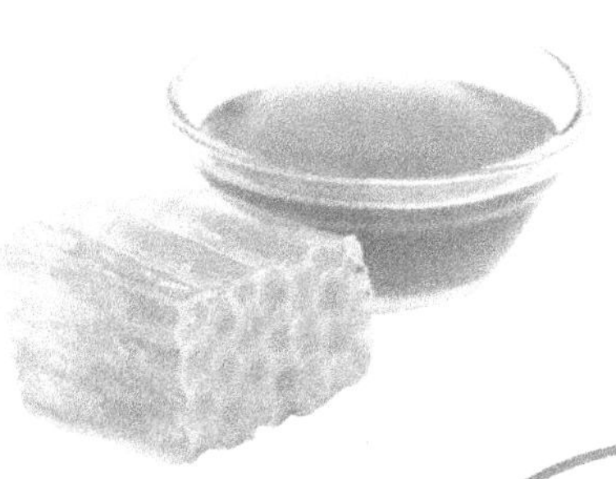

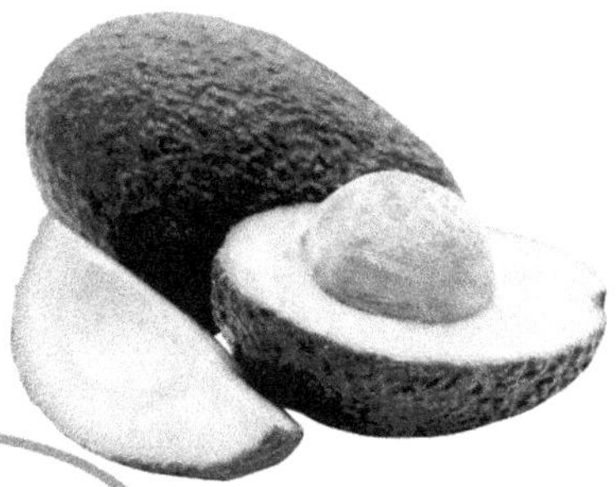

HONEY :

- Honey is a natural humectant, which means it attracts and retains moisture, thus keeping hair hydrated and moisturized.
- Honey is rich in antioxidants and minerals that can stimulate blood flow to the scalp, promoting hair growth.
- Honey is packed with vitamins and minerals that can strengthen hair, making it less prone to breakage.

AVOCADO :

- Avocado can add shine to hair, making it look healthy and lustrous.
- Avocado is a good source of biotin, a B-vitamin that is essential for hair growth.
- Avocado can help to reduce frizz and flyaways, leaving hair looking sleek and smooth.
- Avocado can be used as a natural hair conditioner, making hair soft, smooth and easy to manage.

Coffee & Coconut Oil Cellulite Scrub

- Mix 1/4 cup of ground coffee with 1/4 cup of coconut oil.

- Use the mixture to gently massage any areas of cellulite on your body.

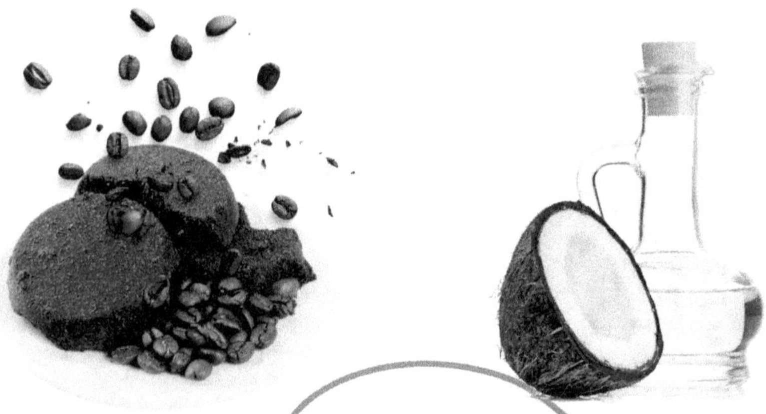

COFFEE :

- The granules in coffee grounds can act as a natural exfoliant, helping to remove dead skin cells and reveal smoother brighter skin.
- Caffeine in coffee can stimulate blood flow, which can help to reduce puffiness and dark circles around the eyes.
- The caffeine in coffee can help to reduce the appearance of cellulite by stimulating blood flow and breaking down fat cells.

COCONUT OIL :

- Coconut oil is a natural emollient, which means it can penetrate the skin and moisturize it from within.
- The fatty acids in coconut oil can improve skin elasticity, making the skin look firmer and more youthful.
- Coconut oil has antimicrobial properties that can help to promote wound healing, and also can be used as a natural sunscreen.

Rosewater & Witch Hazel Facial Mist

- Mix 1/4 cup of rosewater with 1 tablespoon of witch hazel.

- Store the mixture in a spray bottle and use as a refreshing facial mist throughout the day

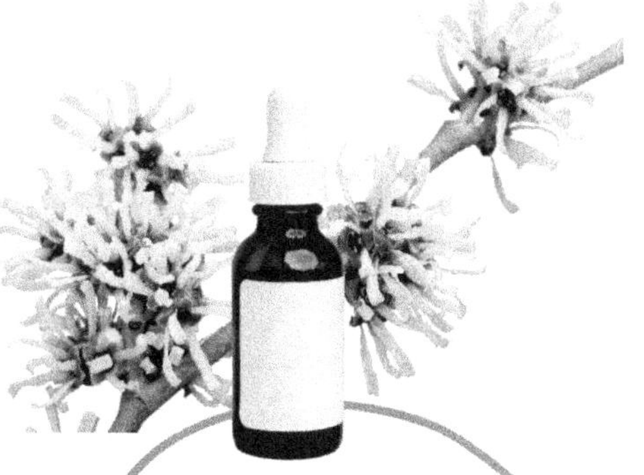

WITCH HAZEL :

- Witch hazel has natural anti-inflammatory properties that can help to reduce redness and inflammation in the skin.
- Witch hazel is an astringent, meaning it can help to tighten and tone the skin, which can be beneficial for oily or acne-prone skin.
- Witch hazel can be used as a toner, it can help to balance the skin's pH, tighten pores and remove excess oil.
- Witch hazel can be used as a natural cleanser, it can help to remove dirt, oil, and makeup without stripping the skin of its natural oils.

Lemon & Baking Soda Teeth Whitener

- Mix 1 teaspoon of baking soda with 1 teaspoon of freshly squeezed lemon juice.
- Use the mixture as a toothpaste to gently whiten your teeth

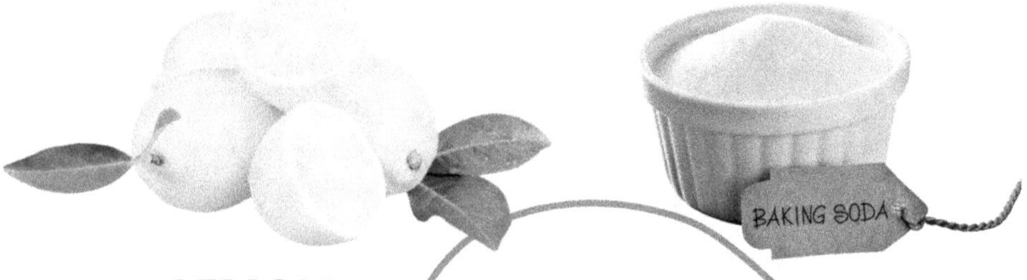

LEMON :

- Help to remove surface stains on the teeth caused by coffee, tea, and tobacco.
- It can help to freshen the breath.
- The acid in lemon juice can help to remove plaque, the sticky film of bacteria that forms on teeth.
- it is important to rinse your mouth well after use, and avoid brushing your teeth with lemon juice regularly as it can erode the enamel.

BAKING SODA :

- Baking soda has mild abrasive properties that can help to gently scrub away surface stains and whiten the teeth.
- Baking soda can neutralize acid in the mouth, which can help to prevent tooth decay and erosion.
- Baking soda can help to neutralize odor-causing bacteria in the mouth, leaving the breath smelling fresh.

Coconut Oil & Lime Cuticle Cream

- Mix 1 tablespoon of coconut oil with 1 teaspoon of freshly squeezed lime juice.

- Apply the mixture to your cuticles to moisturize and strengthen them.

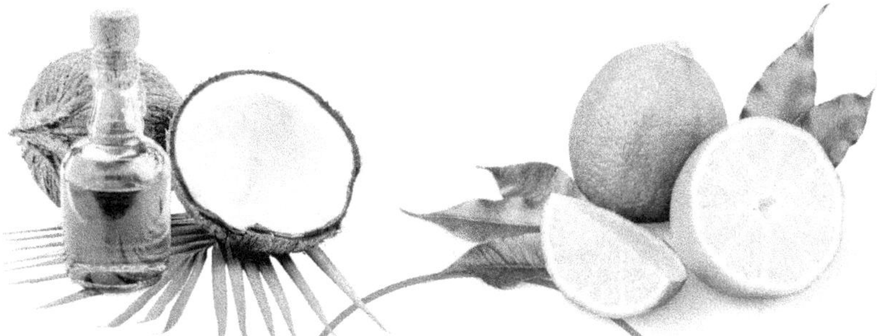

COCONUT OIL:

- It can help to improve blood circulation and promote healthy cuticles.
- It can help to strengthen the nails by providing them with the necessary moisture and nourishment.
- It can help to soften and loosen the cuticles, making them easier to push back.

LIME :

- Can help to exfoliate the cuticles.
- Can help to improve the appearance of dry and cracked cuticles.
- Can help to promote healthy nails.
- Can help to soften the cuticles.
- It can help to strengthen the nails by providing them with the necessary moisture and nourishment.

- Mix 1/4 cup of aloe vera gel with 1 tablespoon of jojoba oil.

- Apply the mixture to your skin after sun exposure to soothe and hydrate it.

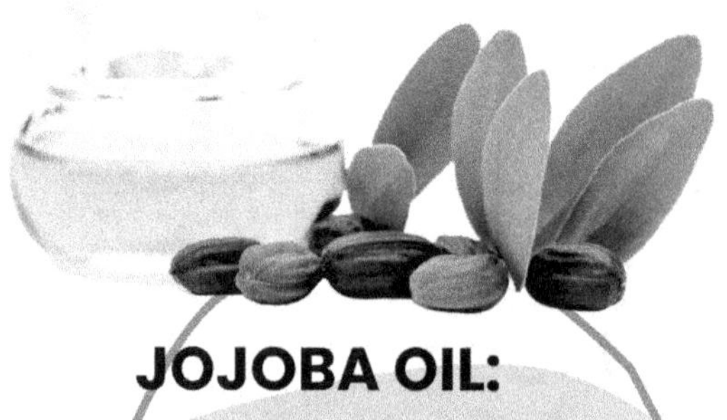

JOJOBA OIL:

- Jojoba oil is a natural emollient, which means it can penetrate the skin and moisturize it from within.
- Jojoba oil is rich in antioxidants that can help to improve the appearance of fine lines and wrinkles by protecting the skin from damage.
- Jojoba oil has antimicrobial properties that can help to reduce the appearance of acne by preventing the growth of bacteria.
- Jojoba oil has anti-inflammatory properties that can help to reduce redness and inflammation in the skin.

Oats & Milk Bath Soak

- Mix 1 cup of rolled oats with 1 cup of milk powder.

- . Add the mixture to a warm bath and soak for 20-30 minutes.

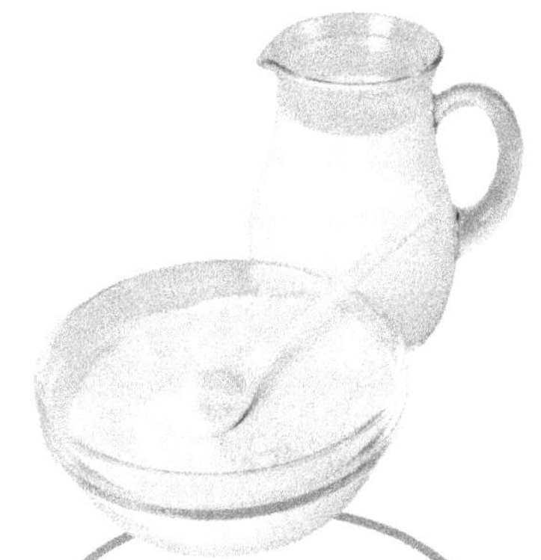

MILK :

- Milk contains lactic acid which is a natural alpha-hydroxy acid (AHA) that helps to moisturize and hydrate the skin.
- The lactic acid in milk can help to improve the appearance of fine lines and wrinkles by promoting collagen production, which can improve skin elasticity.
- Milk can be used as a natural cleanser, it can help to remove dirt, oil, and makeup without stripping the skin of its natural oils.
- Milk contains a compound called "lactose" which can help to lighten the skin, reducing the appearance of dark spots and blemishes.

Lemon and Sugar Hand Scrub

- Mix 1/4 cup of sugar with 1 tablespoon of freshly squeezed lemon juice.

- Use the mixture to gently exfoliate your hands.

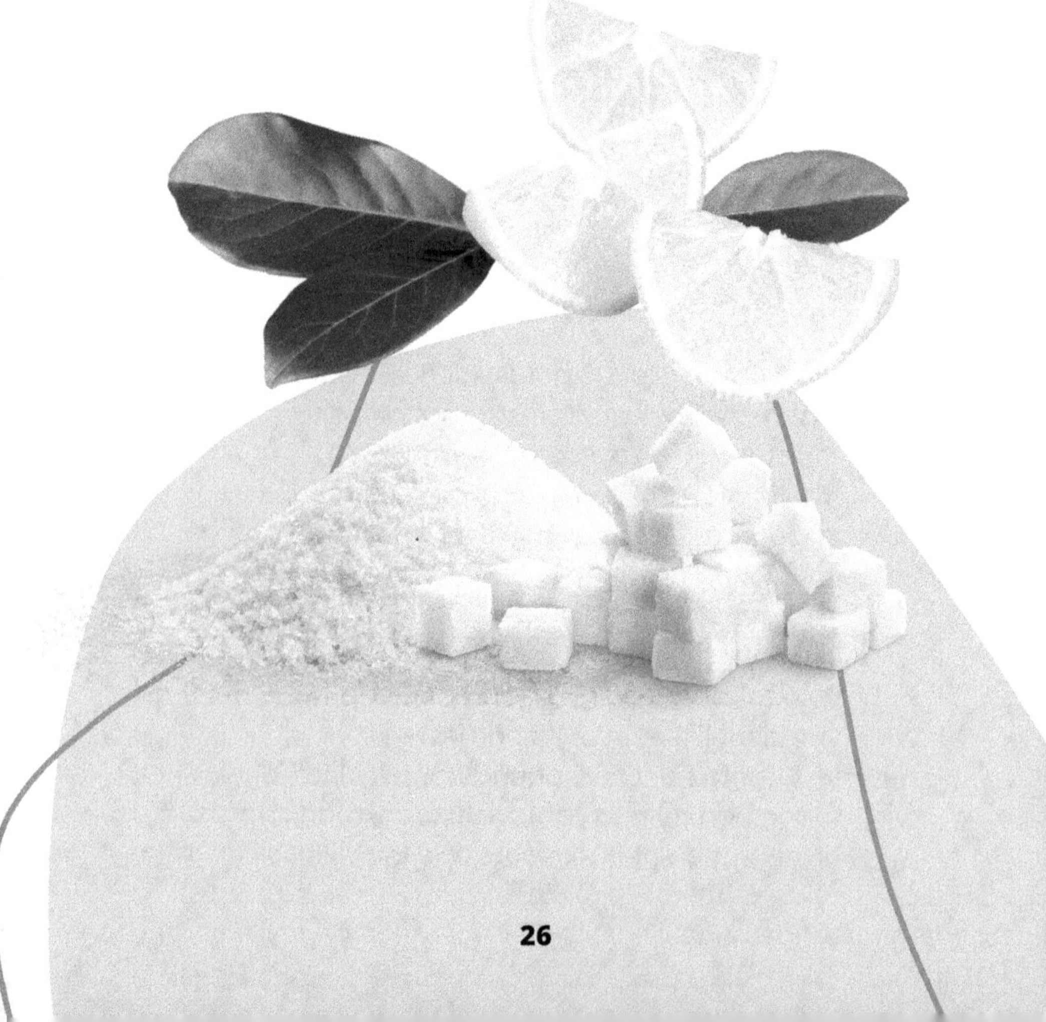

Green Tea & Lemon Juice Eye Cream

- Steep 1 green tea bag in 1/4 cup of hot water for 5 minutes.

- Remove the tea bag and let the tea cool. Mix the tea with 1 tablespoon of lemon juice.

- Apply the mixture to the under-eye area to reduce puffiness and dark circles.

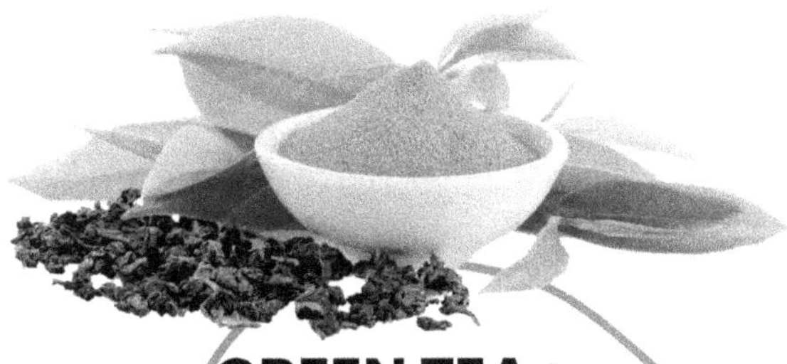

GREEN TEA :

- Green tea is rich in antioxidants such as catechins, which can protect the skin from damage caused by free radicals and improve the overall health and appearance of the skin.
- Green tea has anti-inflammatory properties that can help to soothe irritated skin and reduce redness and puffiness.
- Green tea can help to protect the skin from the signs of aging, such as fine lines and wrinkles, by reducing inflammation and promoting collagen production.
- Green tea contains compounds that can help to protect the skin from the harmful effects of UV radiation.

Honey & Cinnamon Lip Balm

- Mix 1 teaspoon of honey with 1/4 teaspoon of cinnamon powder.

- Apply the mixture to your lips to hydrate and plump them.

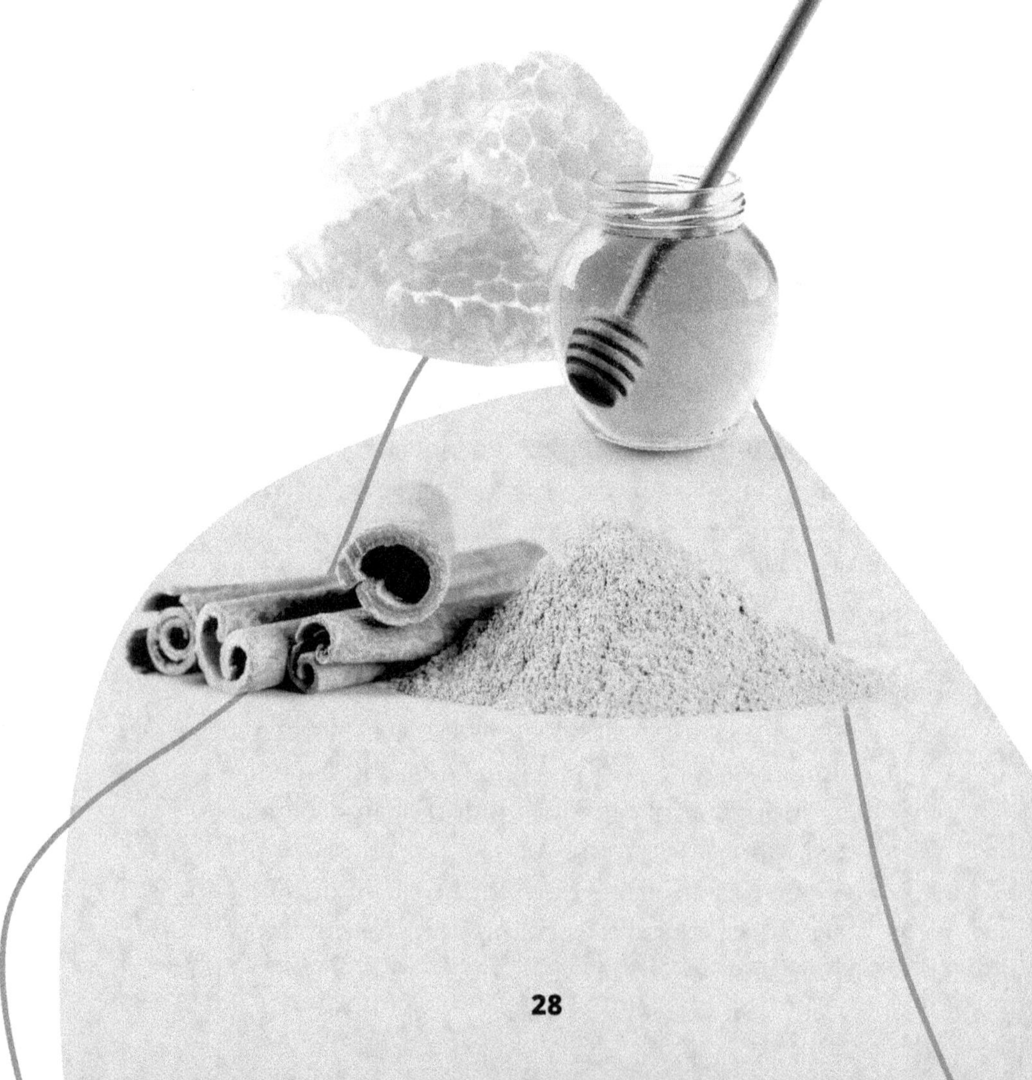

Coconut Oil & Vanilla Bean Hair Mask

- Mix 1/4 cup of coconut oil with 1/2 of a vanilla bean.

- Apply the mixture to your hair and leave on for 30 minutes before rinsing off.

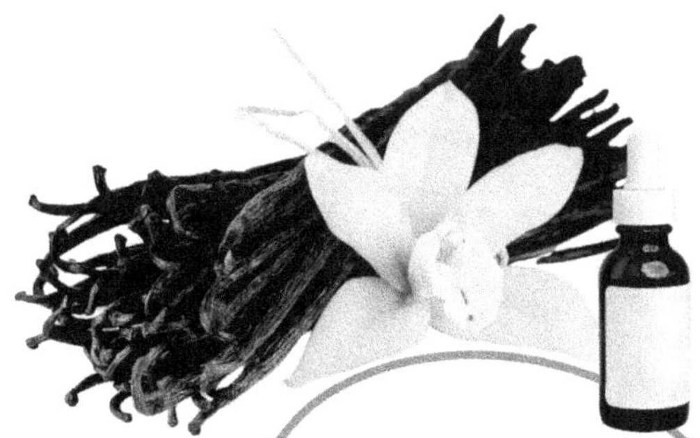

VANILLA BEAN EXTRACT :

- Vanilla has anti-inflammatory properties, which can help to soothe and calm irritated skin.
- Anti-bacterial. Vanilla has been used to reduce skin infections and in wound healing.
- Vanilla Bean Extract contains Vanillin, a polyphenol with powerful anti-oxidant properties.
- Anti-oxidants help to protect against free radical damage and the effects of environmental stresses on the skin.
- Vanilla also contains B vitamins, including niacin, thiamin, riboflavin, vitamin B6, and pantothenic acid. All of which help to maintain healthy looking skin.

Aloe Vera & Cucumber Face Mask

- Mix 1/4 cup of aloe vera gel with 1/4 cup of mashed cucumber.

- Apply the mixture to your face and leave on for 15-20 minutes before rinsing off.

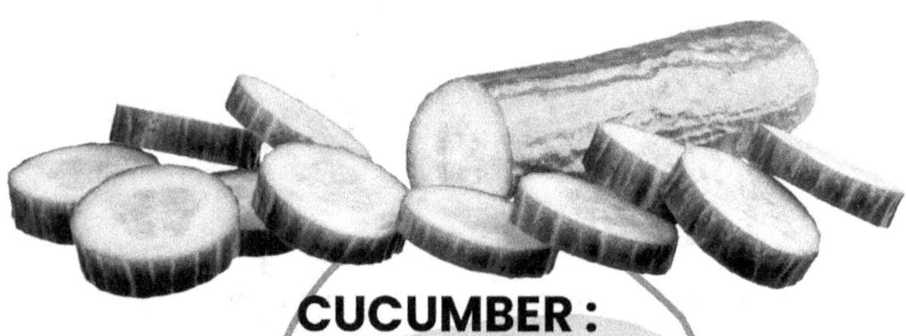

CUCUMBER :

- Cucumbers are made up of mostly water, which makes them an excellent source of hydration for the skin. They can help to soothe dry, irritated skin and improve overall skin tone and texture.
- Cucumbers contain compounds such as cucurbitacins and flavonoids that have anti-inflammatory properties, which can help to reduce redness and puffiness in the skin.
- Cucumbers contain antioxidants such as vitamin C and caffeic acid, which can help to protect the skin from damage caused by free radicals and reduce the appearance of fine lines and wrinkles.

Oatmeal & Honey Body Lotion

- Mix 1/2 cup of oatmeal with 1/4 cup of honey.

- Apply the mixture to your skin as a lotion to moisturize and soothe it.

- Then, rinse it off.

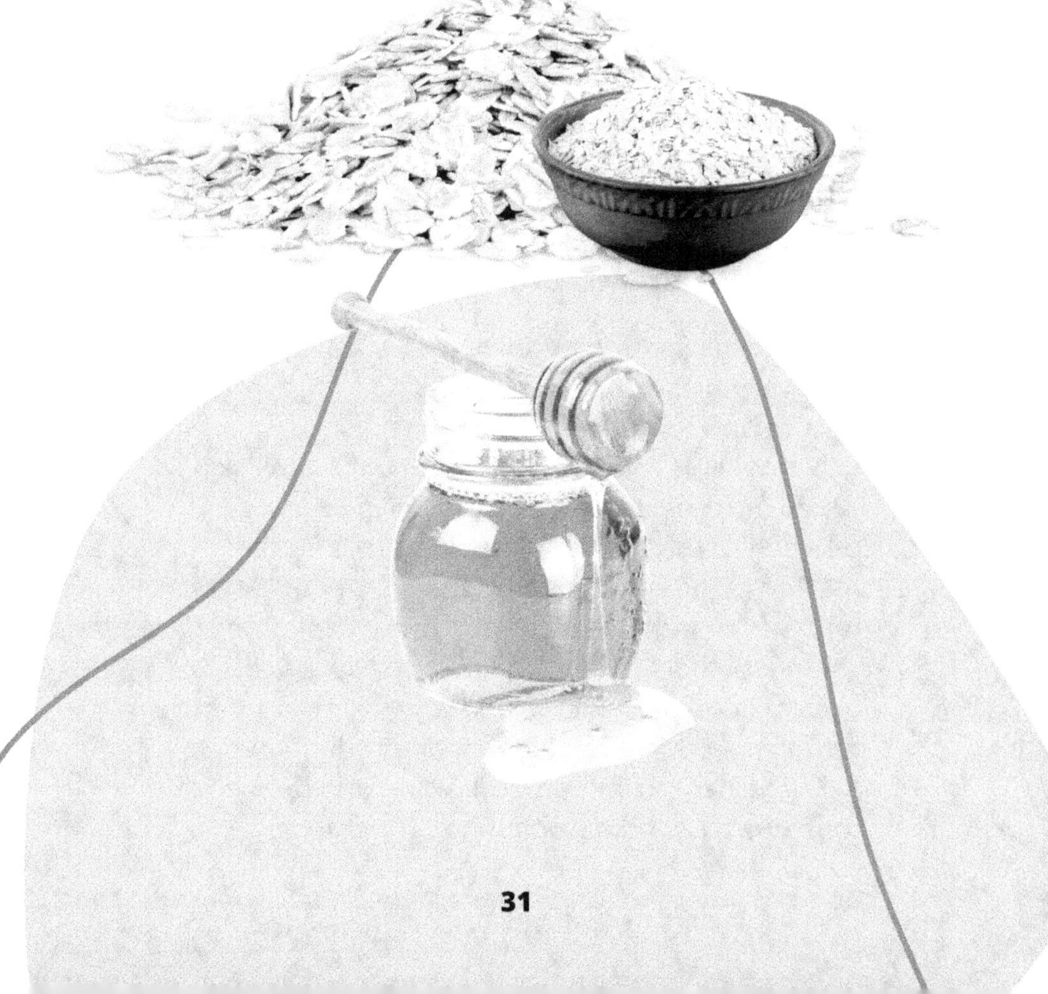

Apple Cider Vinegar & Green Tea Toner

- Mix 1/4 cup of green tea with 1 tablespoon of apple cider vinegar.

- Apply the mixture to your face with a cotton ball or pad.

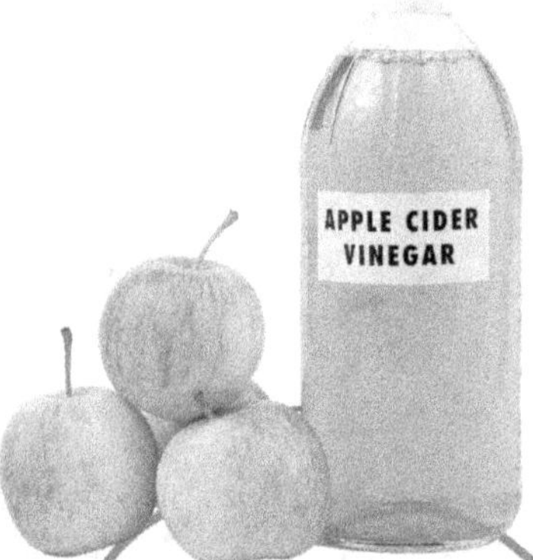

APPLE CIDER VINEGAR:

- ACV contains alpha hydroxy acids (AHAs) which can help to gently exfoliate the skin and improve its texture and tone.
- ACV has a pH level similar to that of healthy skin which can help to balance the skin's pH levels, preventing the growth of bacteria and yeast.
- ACV has antimicrobial properties that can help to kill bacteria that cause acne and reduce inflammation.
- The acetic acid in ACV can help to reduce the appearance of fine lines and wrinkles by tightening the skin and increasing collagen production.
- ACV can help to lighten dark spots and uneven skin tone due to its mild exfoliating properties.

Rosehip Oil & Jojoba Oil Night Cream

- Mix 1 tablespoon of rosehip oil with 1 tablespoon of jojoba oil.

- Apply the mixture to your face as a night cream to nourish and hydrate your skin while you sleep.

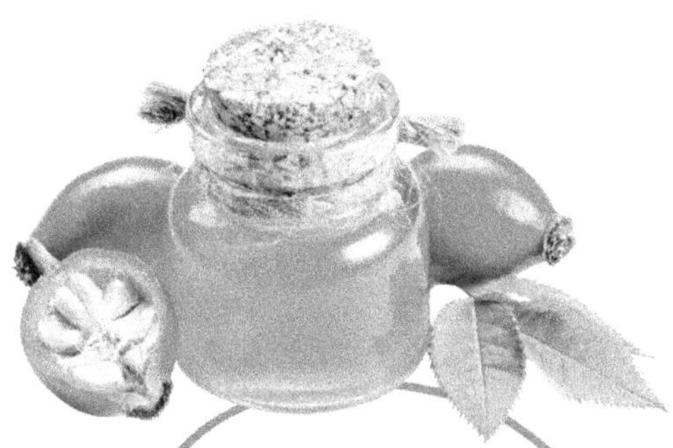

ROSEHIP OIL :

- Rosehip oil is rich in fatty acids, which can help to deeply moisturize and hydrate the skin.
- Rosehip oil is rich in essential fatty acids, which can help to repair and heal damaged skin. It also has anti-inflammatory properties that can help to soothe irritated skin.
- Rosehip oil has been traditionally used to reduce the appearance of scars, including acne scars.
- Rosehip oil is high in antioxidants, such as vitamin C and beta-carotene, which can help to protect the skin from damage caused by free radicals and reduce the appearance of fine lines and wrinkles.
- Rosehip oil can help to even out the skin tone and reduce the appearance of dark spots and hyperpigmentation.

Yogurt & Lemon Juice Facial Cleanser

- Mix 1/4 cup of plain yogurt with 1 tablespoon of freshly squeezed lemon juice.

- Apply the mixture to your face and massage in circular motions for 1-2 minutes before rinsing off.

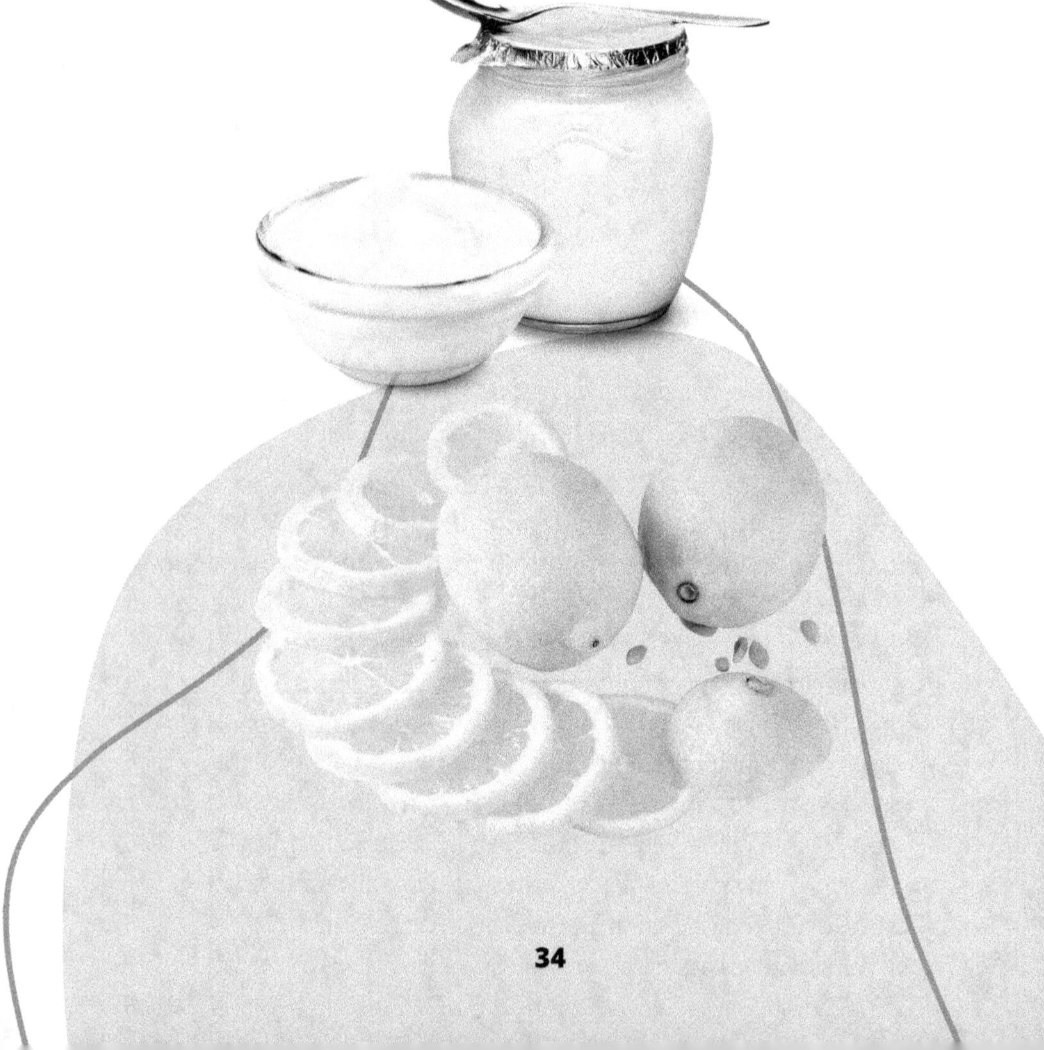

Coconut Oil & Coffee Body Scrub

- Mix 1/4 cup of coconut oil with 1/4 cup of ground coffee.

- Use the mixture to gently exfoliate your skin in the shower.

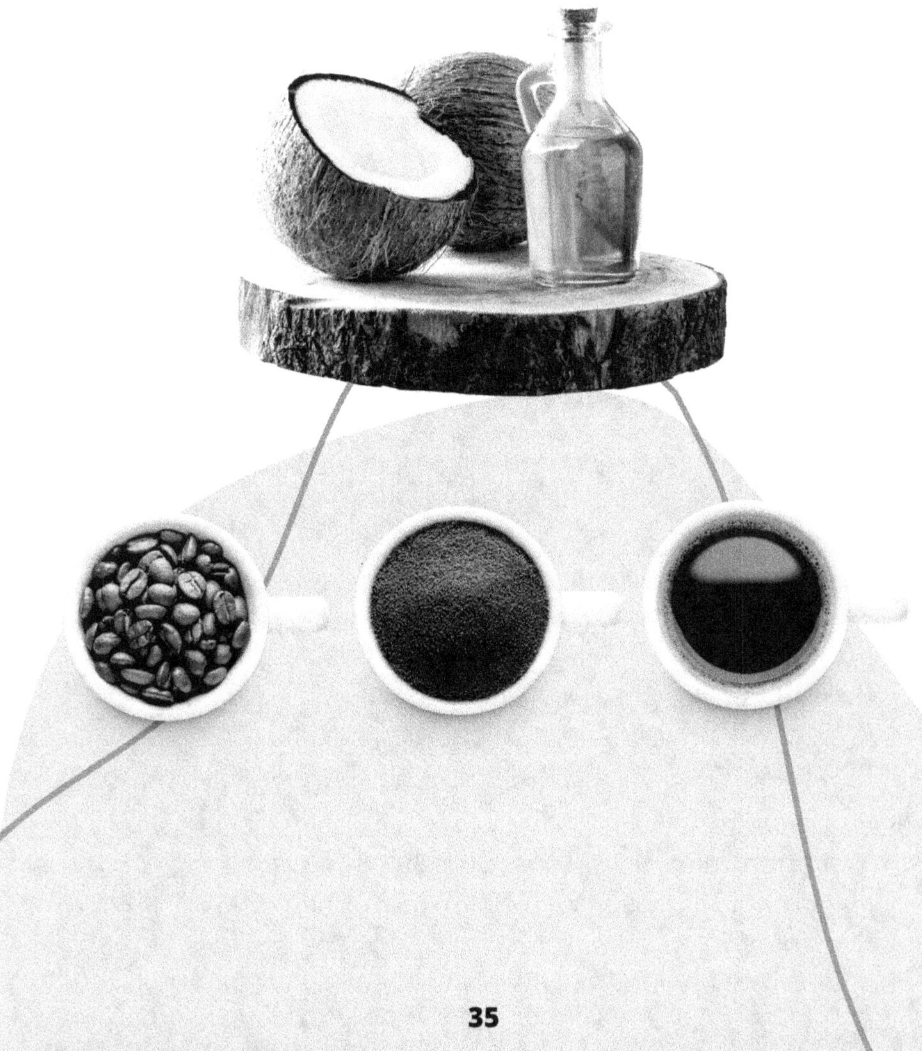

Aloe Vera & Peppermint Lip Balm

- Mix 1 tablespoon of aloe vera gel with 1 drop of peppermint essential oil.

- Apply the mixture to your lips to hydrate and plump them.

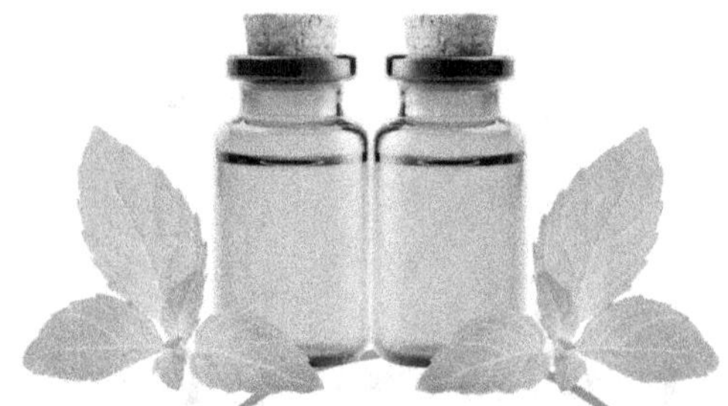

PEPPERMINT ESSENTIAL OIL :

- Peppermint oil is a natural emollient that can help to hydrate and moisturize the lips, making them softer and smoother.
- Peppermint oil has a cooling and soothing effect on the lips, which can help to reduce inflammation and redness.
- Peppermint oil has a refreshing and stimulating effect on the lips, which can help to improve blood circulation and give the lips a healthy, plump appearance.
- Peppermint oil has a natural SPF that can help to protect the lips from the harmful effects of UV radiation.

Lavender & Epsom Salt Bath Soak

- Mix 1 cup of Epsom salt with 10 drops of lavender essential oil.

- Add the mixture to a warm bath and soak for 20-30 minutes.

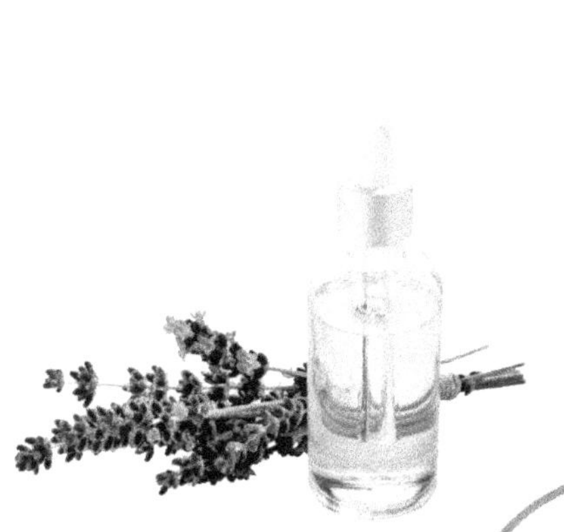

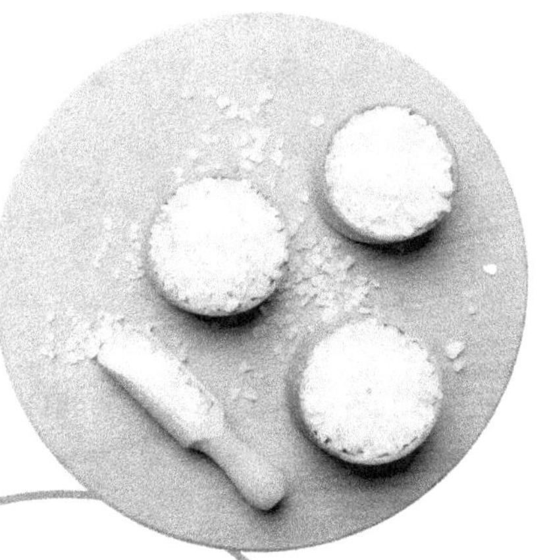

LAVENDER :

- Lavender oil has anti-inflammatory properties that can help to soothe irritated skin, reduce redness and calm skin conditions such as eczema and psoriasis.
- Lavender oil is rich in antioxidants which can help to protect the skin from damage caused by free radicals and reduce the appearance of fine lines and wrinkles.

EPSOM SALT:

- It can help to remove dead skin cells and impurities, leaving the skin feeling refreshed and rejuvenated.
- It can help to draw out toxins and impurities from the skin, which can improve the overall health and appearance of the skin.
- It can help to relax muscles and reduce pain and soreness, making it a popular choice for people with conditions such as arthritis.

Take Care of Your Skin

We have learned about the various benefits of natural ingredients for our skin, and how to make our own skincare products at home.

From honey and turmeric face masks to avocado and banana face scrubs, we have explored a wide variety of recipes that can help to improve the overall health and appearance of our skin.

We hope that these recipes have helped you to achieve a natural and radiant glow and that you will continue to use them in the
future.

As we come to the end of this
book, we want to remind you
that skincare is an ongoing process
and it's important to take care of your
 skin on a daily basis.

Eating a healthy diet, staying hydrated, and getting enough sleep are all important aspects of maintaining healthy skin. Additionally, it's important to protect your skin from the sun by using sunscreen and wearing protective clothing.

We hope that this book has been informative and helpful to you, and that you will continue to explore the world of natural skincare. Remember, nature has provided us with everything we need to achieve beautiful, healthy skin.

With the right ingredients and a little bit of creativity, you can create your own natural skincare products that will leave your skin looking and feeling its best.

Thank you for reading "Nature's Secret to Beautiful Skin: 35 DIY Skincare Recipes for a Natural and Radiant Glowing" and we hope you have a great time experimenting with the recipes provided in the book.

NATHALIE WOODS

Bibliography

"The Complete Book of Essential Oils and Aromatherapy" by Valerie Ann Worwood

"Herbal Beauty: 100 Natural Recipes for a Radiant You" by Julie Gabriel

"The Green Beauty Guide: Your Essential Resource to Organic and Natural Skin Care, Hair Care, Makeup, and Fragrances" by Julie Gabriel

"Organic Body Care Recipes: 175 Homemade Herbal Formulas for Glowing Skin & Hair, Relaxing & Rejuvenating" by Stephanie Tourles

"The Natural Beauty Solution: Unlock the Power of Natural Ingredients for a Beautiful, Healthy You" by Laura Rudoe

"The Skincare Bible: Your No-Nonsense Guide to Great Skin" by Dr. Anjali Mahto

"The Little Book of Skincare: Korean Beauty Secrets for Healthy, Glowing Skin" by Charlotte Cho

"The Beauty of Dirty Skin: The Surprising Science of Looking and Feeling Radiant from the Inside Out" by Dr. Whitney Bowe

"The DIY Skincare Revolution: A Beginner's Guide to Making Your Own Natural and Organic Skincare Products" by Susan D. Bratton

"The Skin Type Solution: A Revolutionary Guide to Your Best Skin Ever" by Leslie Baumann, MD